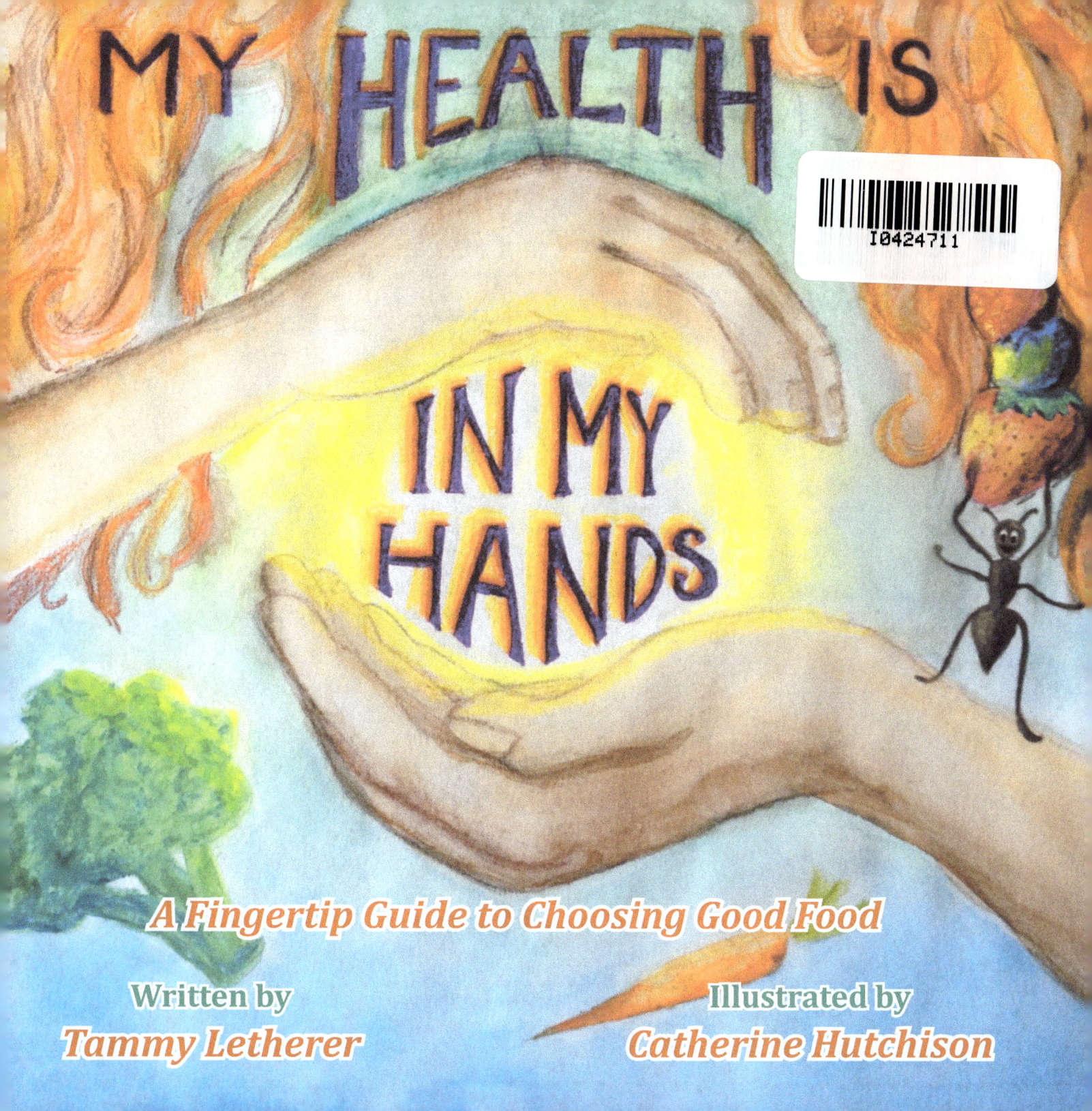

MY HEALTH IS IN MY HANDS

A Fingertip Guide to Choosing Good Food

Written by
Tammy Letherer

Illustrated by
Catherine Hutchison

Balboa Press books may be ordered through booksellers or by contacting:

Balboa Press
A Division of Hay House
1663 Liberty Drive
Bloomington, IN 47403
www.balboapress.com
1 (877) 407-4847

ISBN: 978-1-4525-1618-9 (sc)
ISBN: 978-1-4525-1619-6 (e)

Library of Congress Control Number: 2014909849

Printed in the United States of America.

Balboa Press rev. date: 06/25/2014

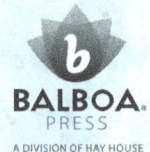

BALBOA.
PRESS
A DIVISION OF HAY HOUSE

My Health is
in My Hands

Hi! I'm hungry.

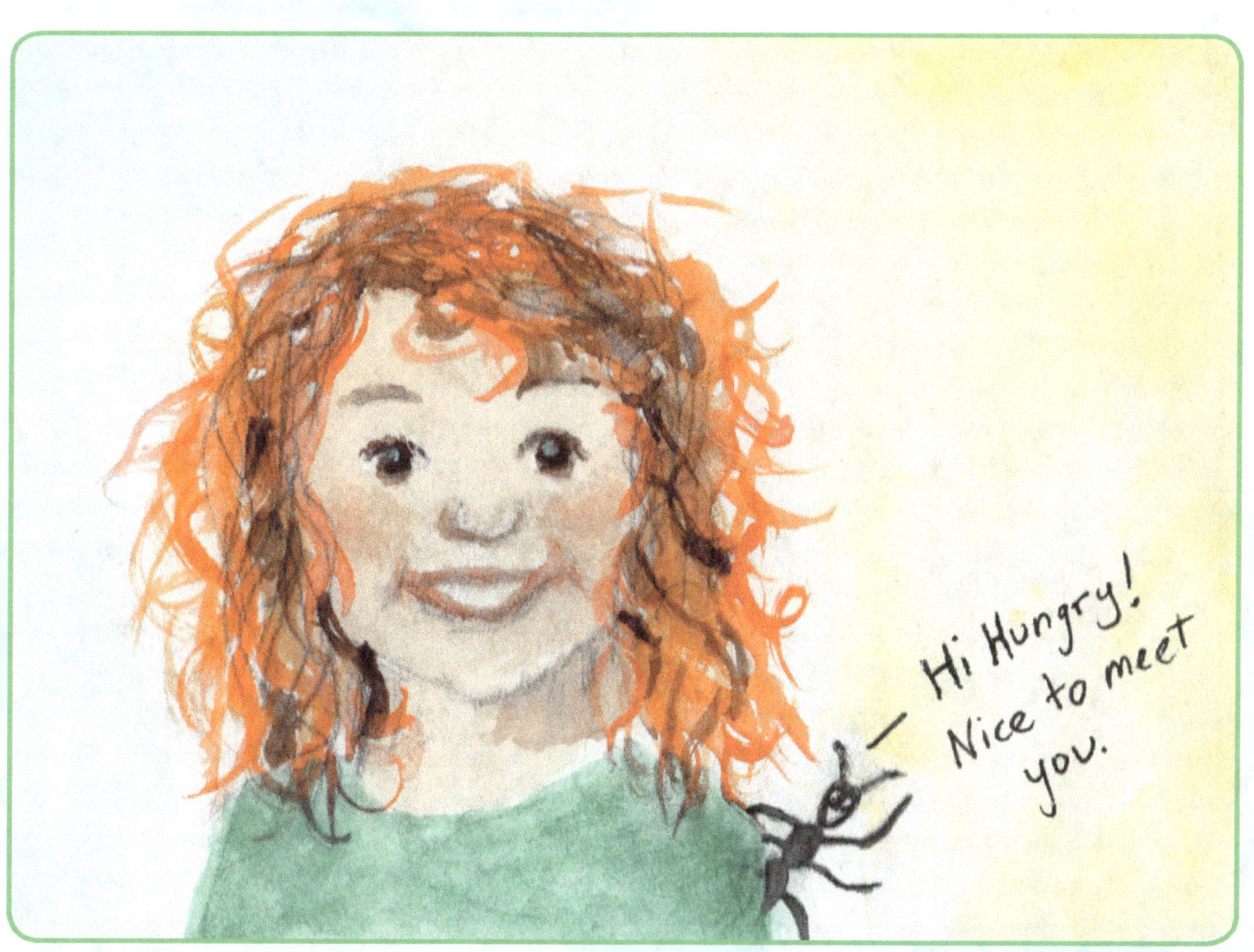

No, silly! That's not my name.

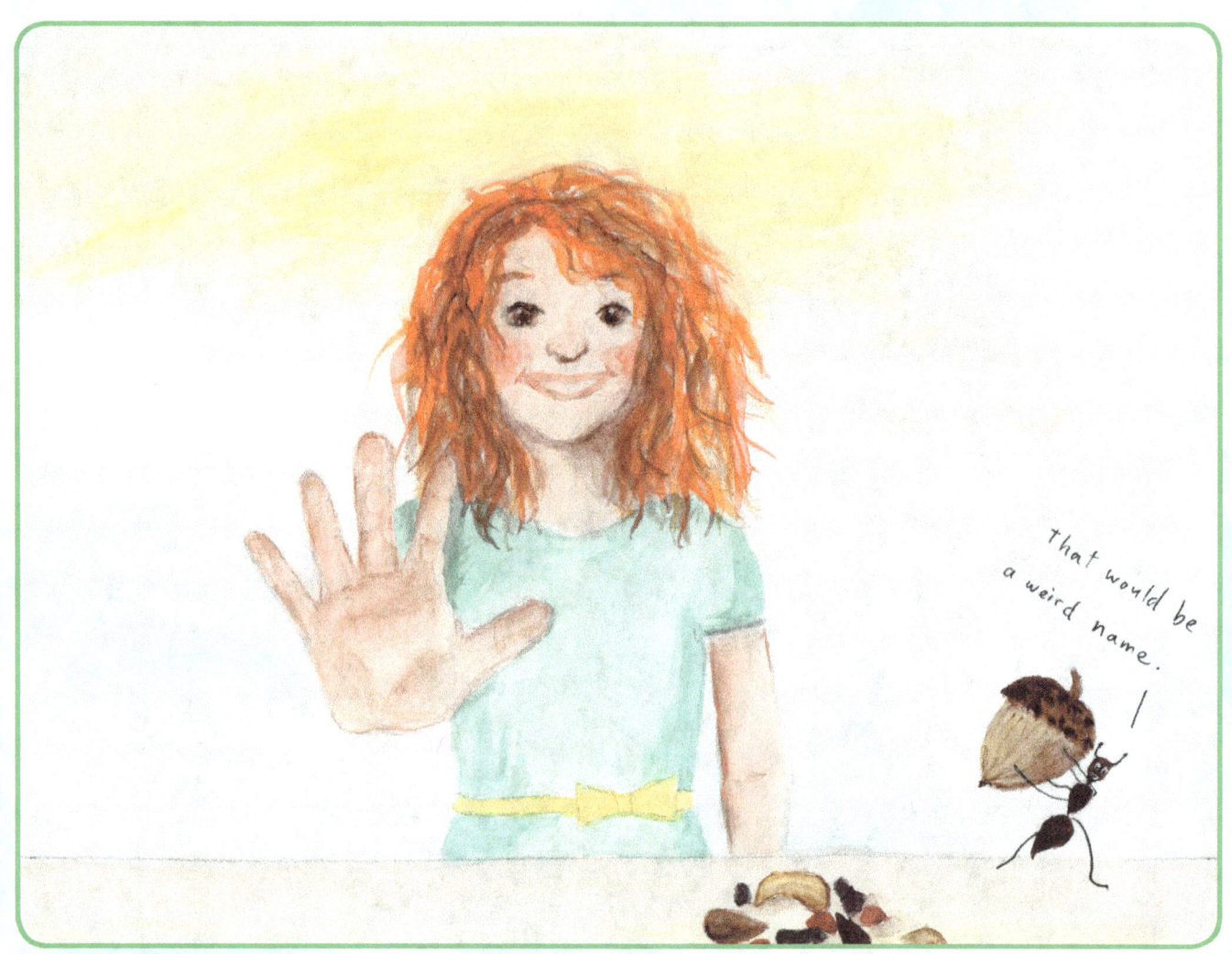

That would be a weird name.

My name is Genevieve. This is my hand. I use my hand to help me choose the best foods to eat.

Thumbs-up foods are *really, really* good for me.

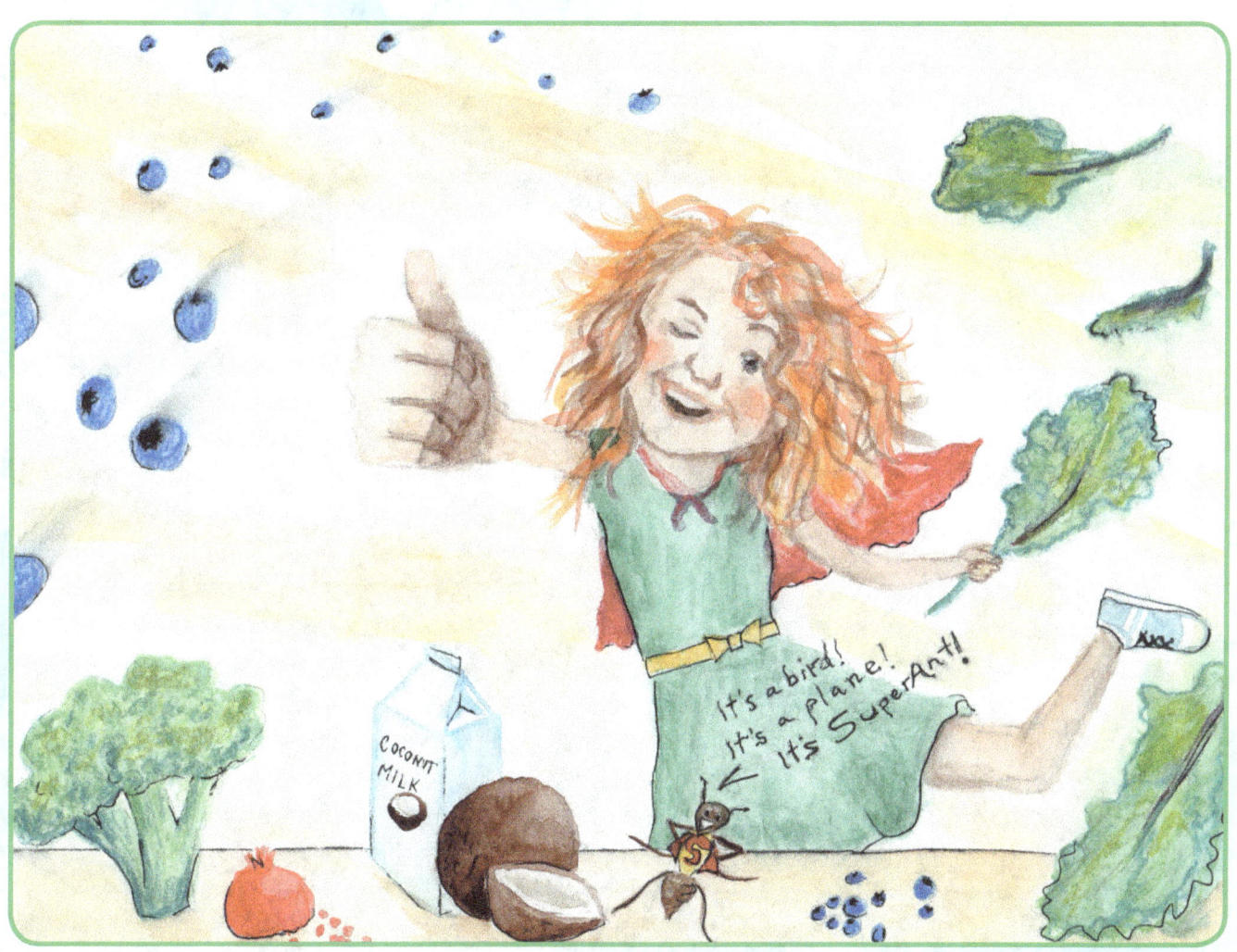

They're so good, they're called SUPER FOODS. My taste buds don't always love them, but my body does.

This is my pointer finger and it points me toward my favorite foods.

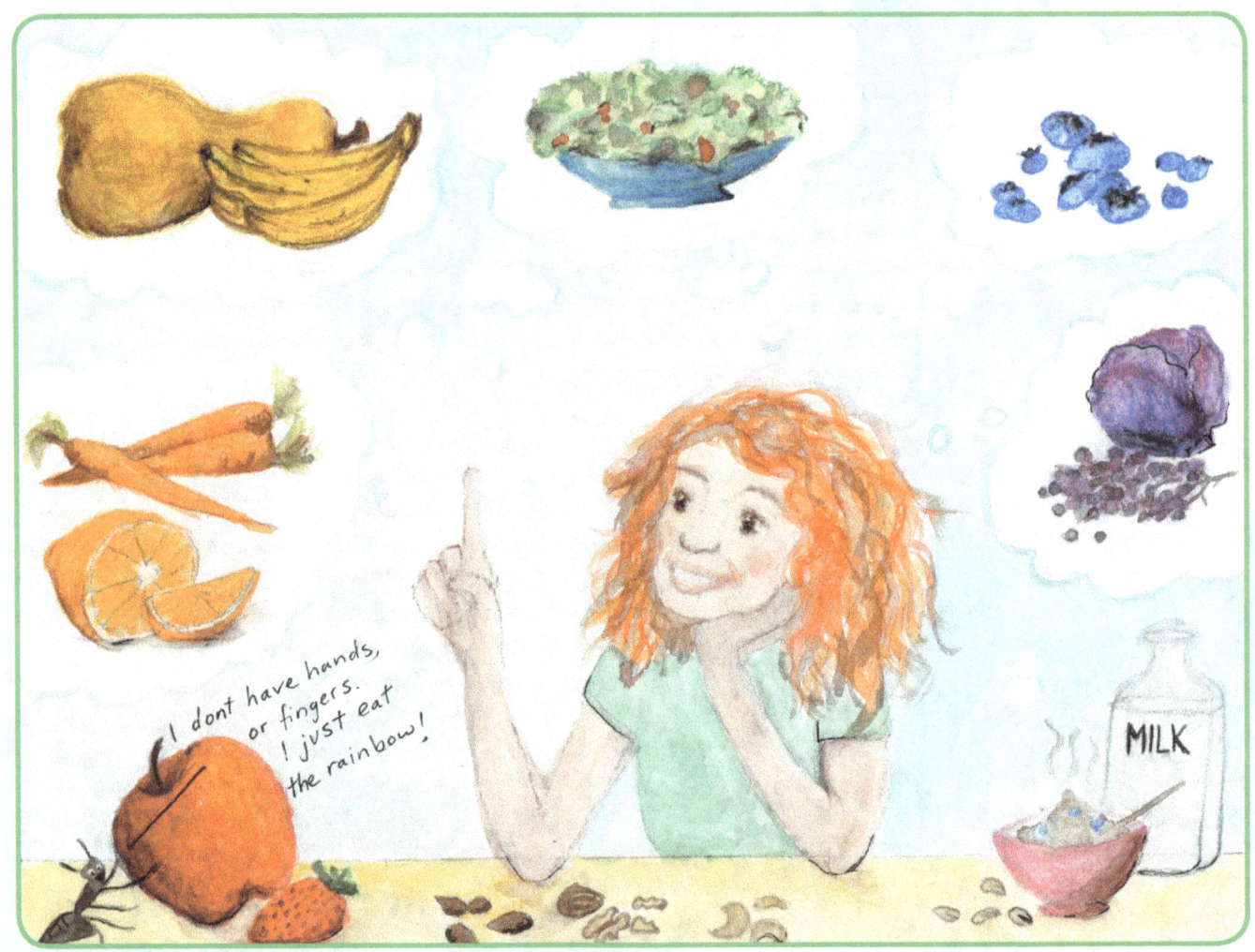

These are foods I eat every day. That's called having good habits.

I named my tallest finger TALL GUY.

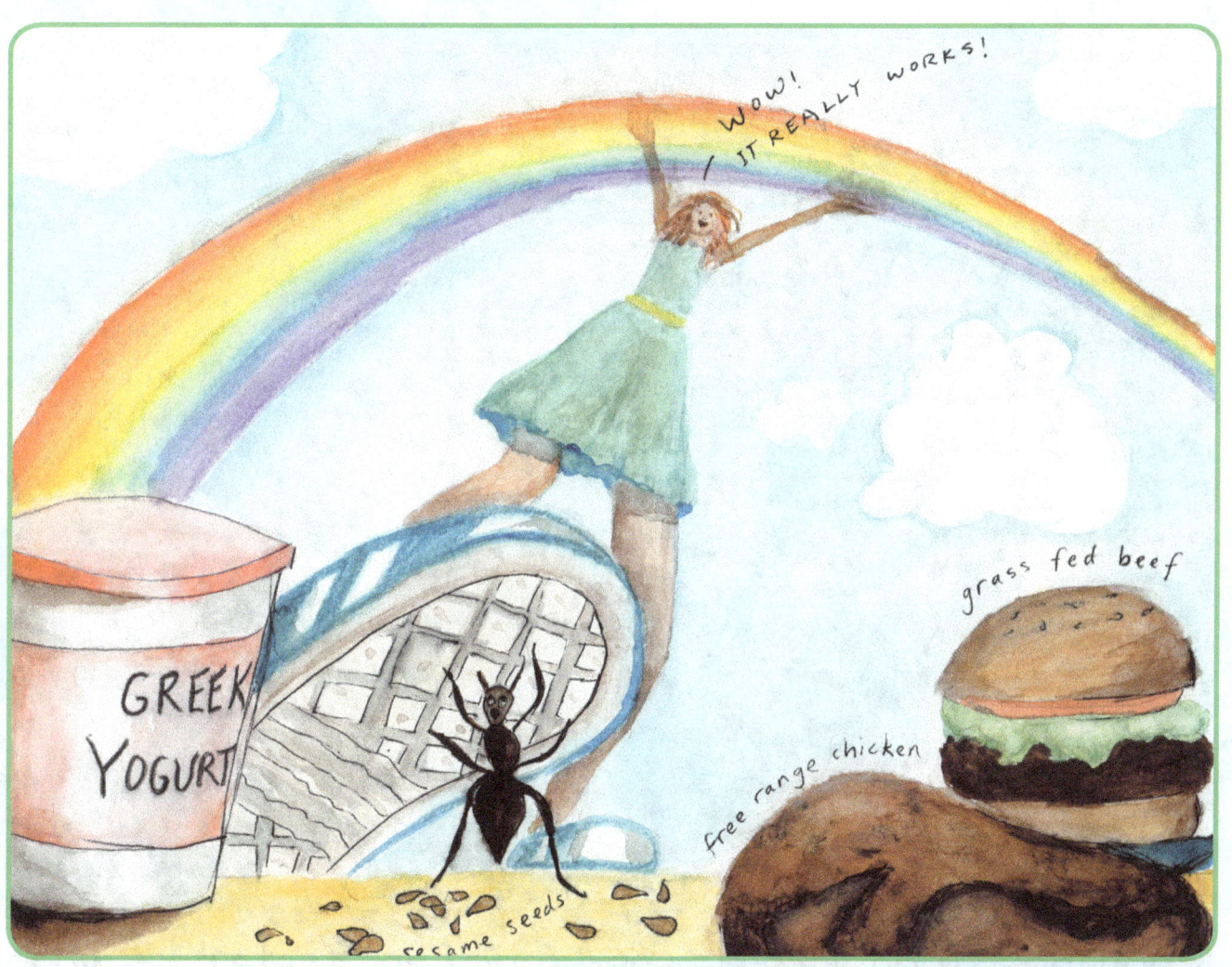

Tall guy reminds me to choose foods that will help me grow big and strong.

My ring finger just loves special, sparkly occasions.

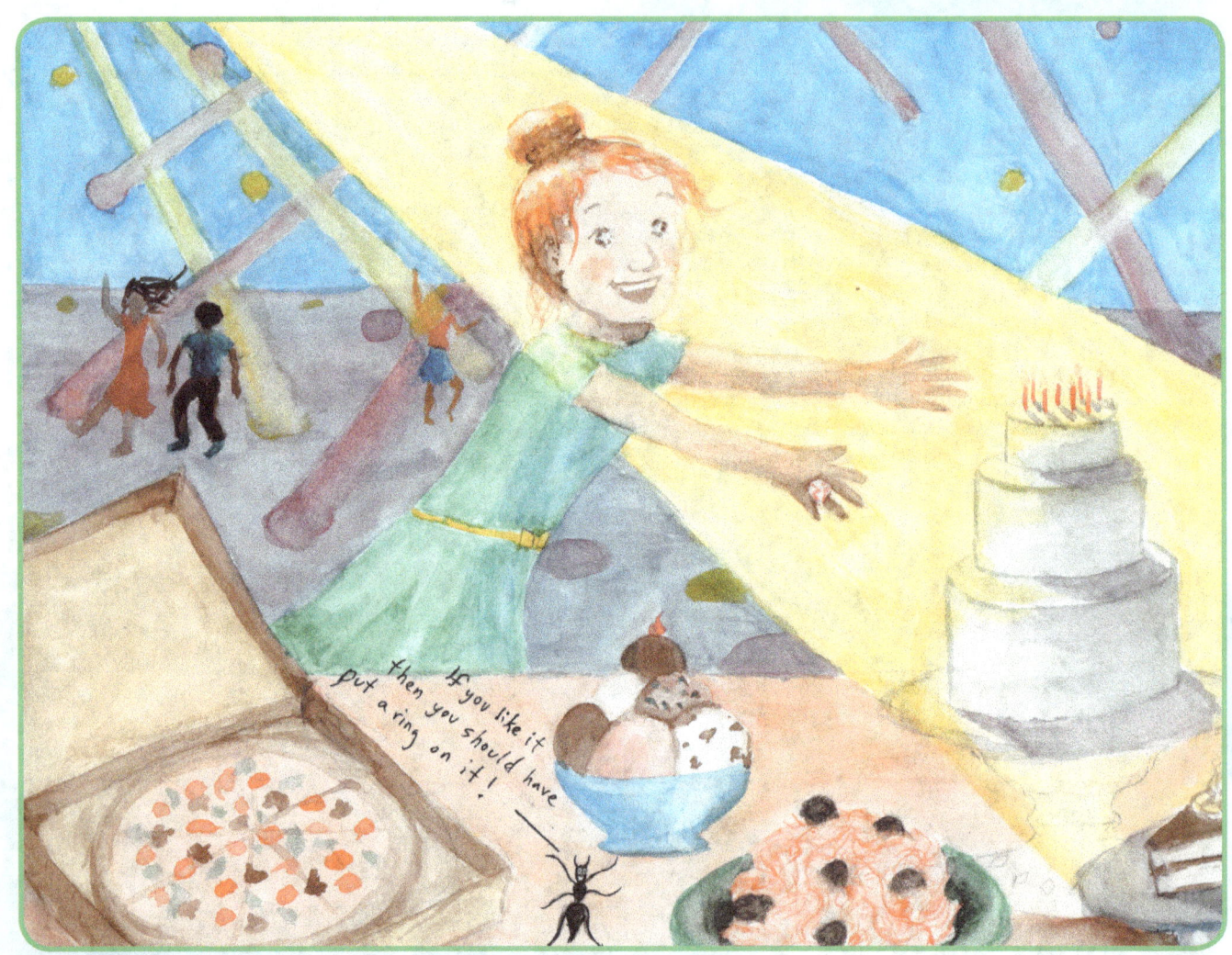

Ring finger foods are rich and fancy and taste best when shared with friends. Having fun is part of being healthy.

Pinky finger foods are not so good for me,

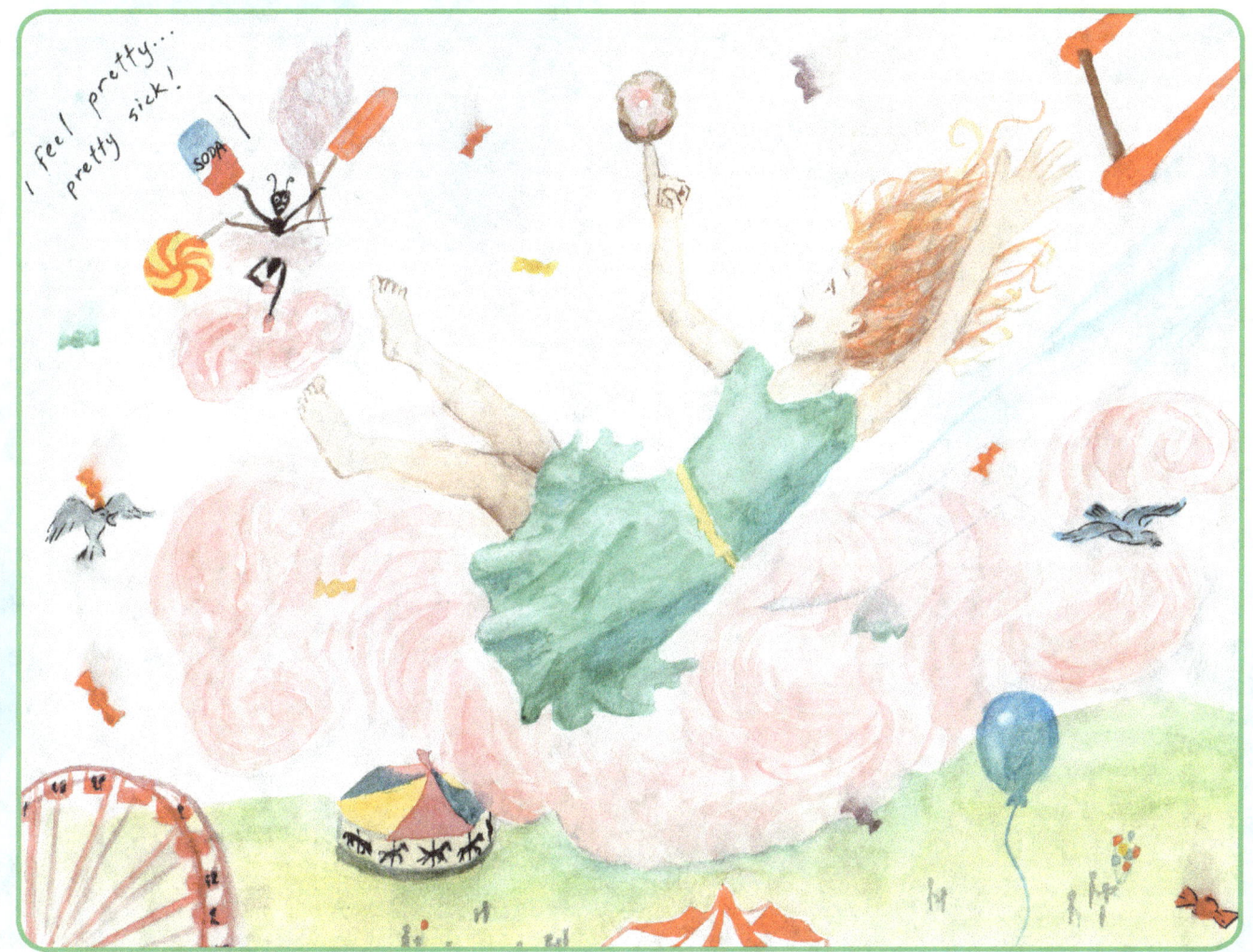

so I eat them only in teeny-weeny, itty-bitty amounts.

Food gives me energy because food is made of energy.

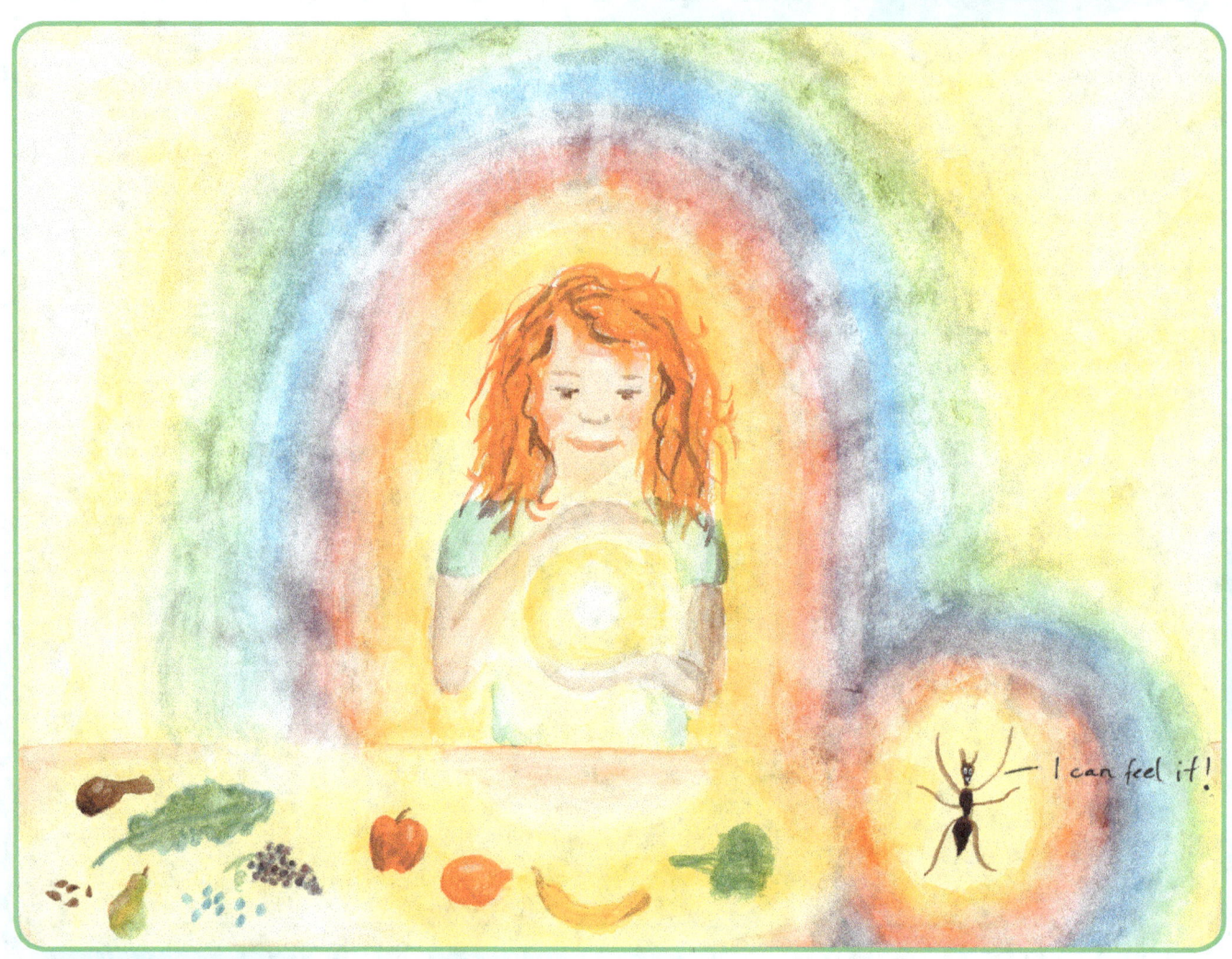

I can feel it!

Go ahead...see if YOU can feel energy with YOUR hands!

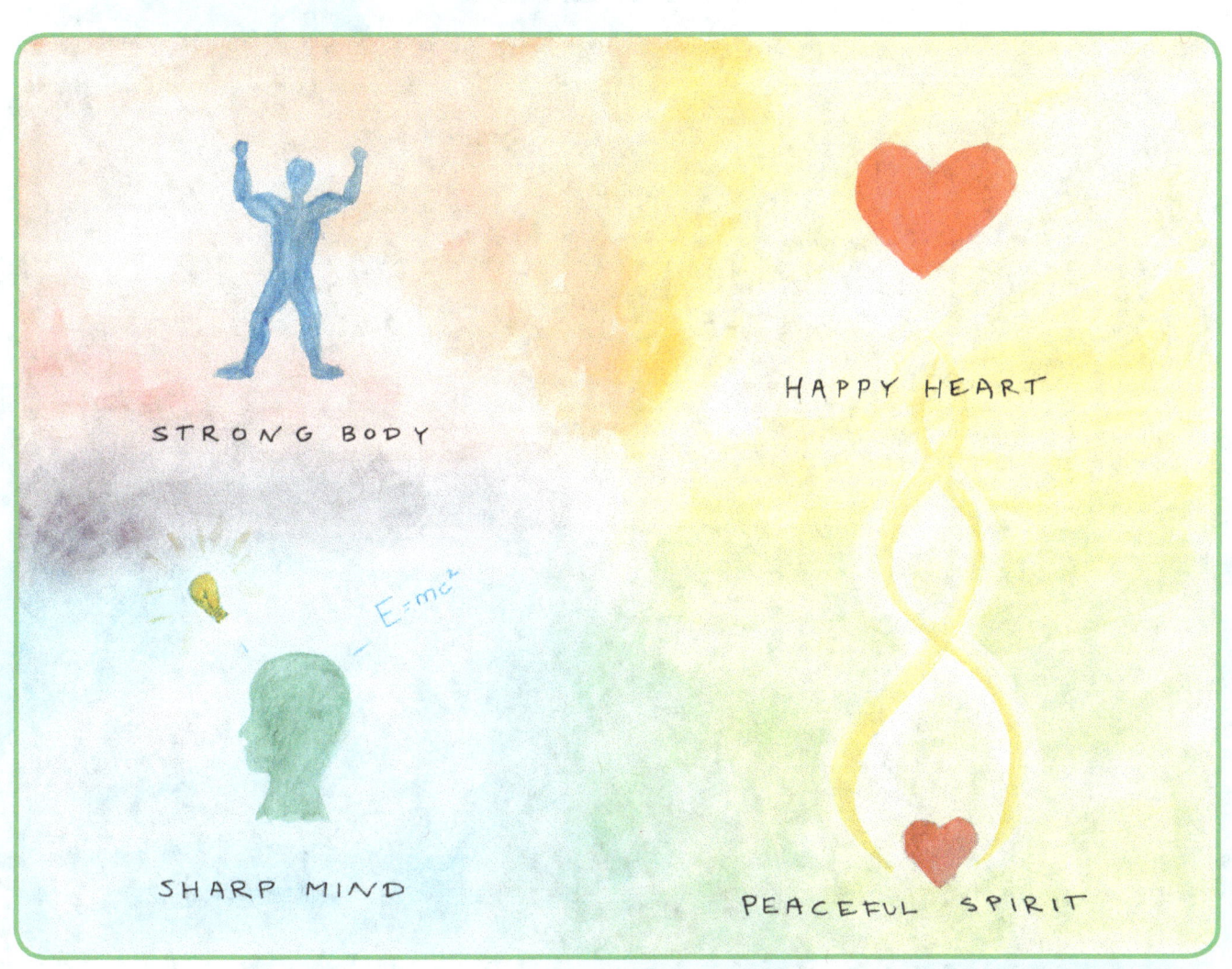

A balanced diet supports a balanced life.

When I'm done choosing my food, I use my hands to give thanks.

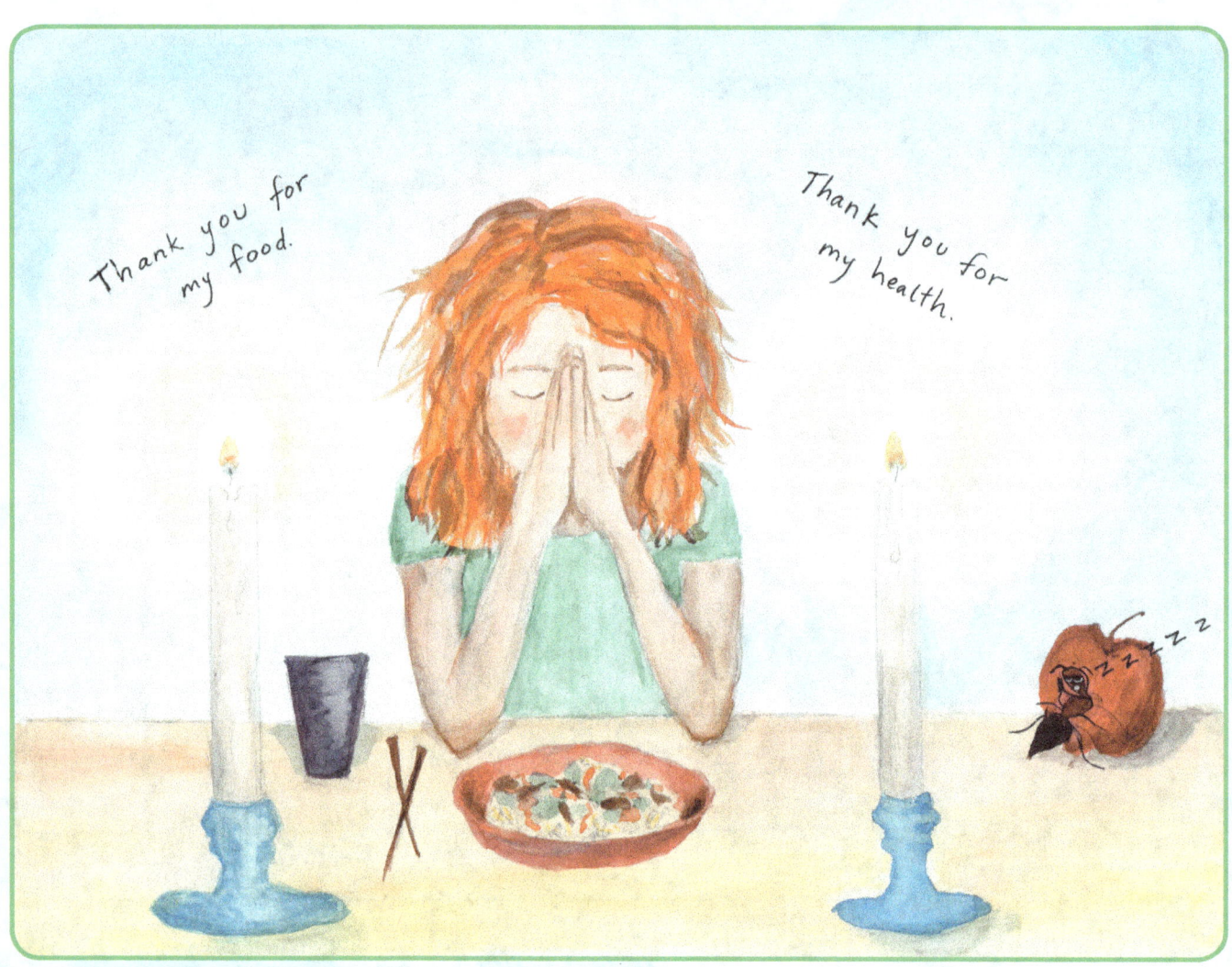

Gratitude makes everything taste better.

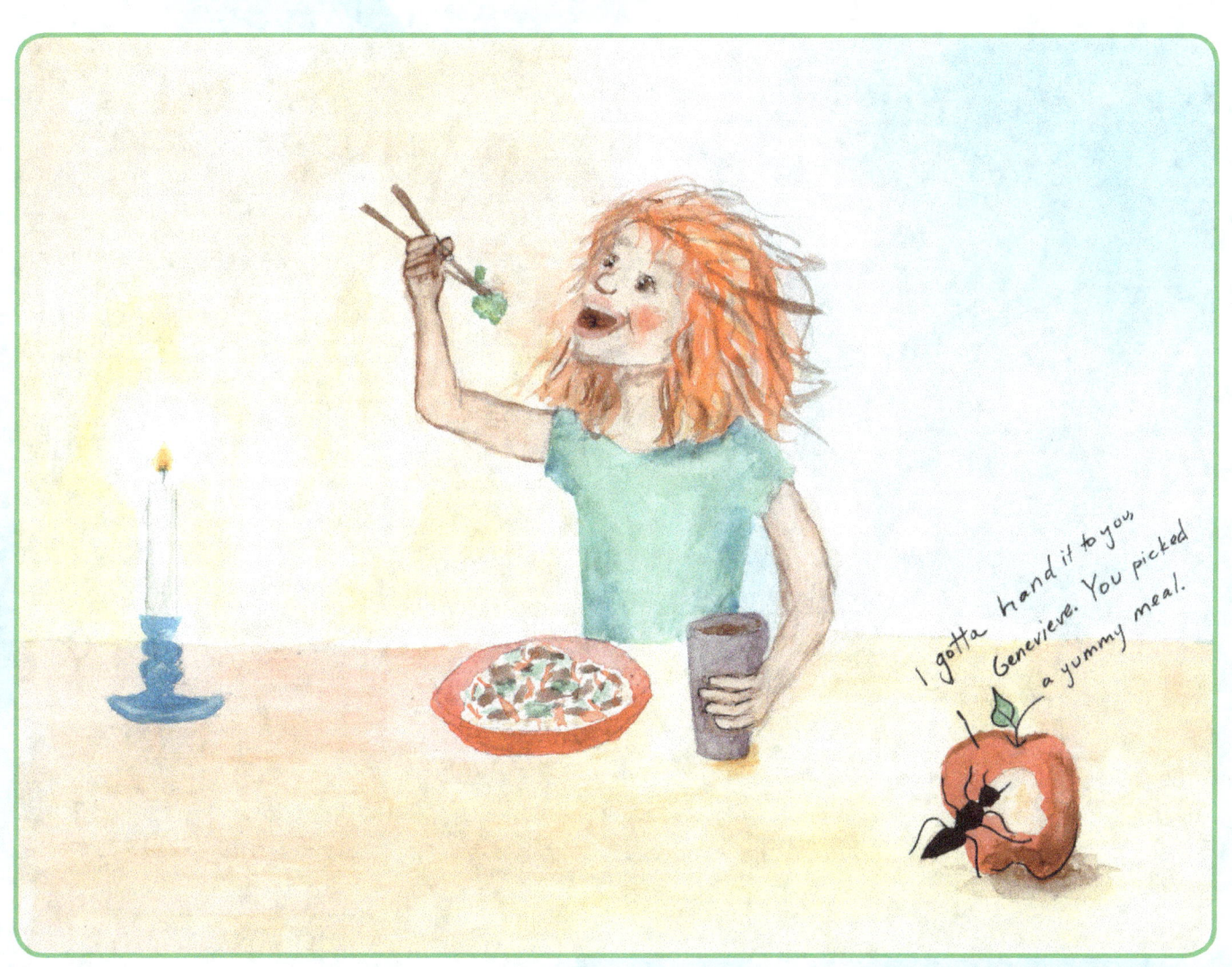

Time to eat!

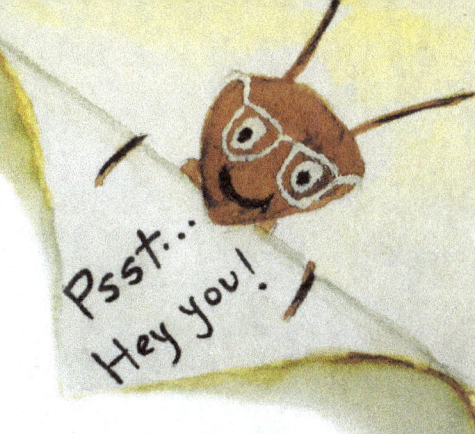
Psst...
Hey you!

- What are 5 foods that make YOUR body feel good?

- What does it mean to eat the rainbow?

- What colors did you eat today?

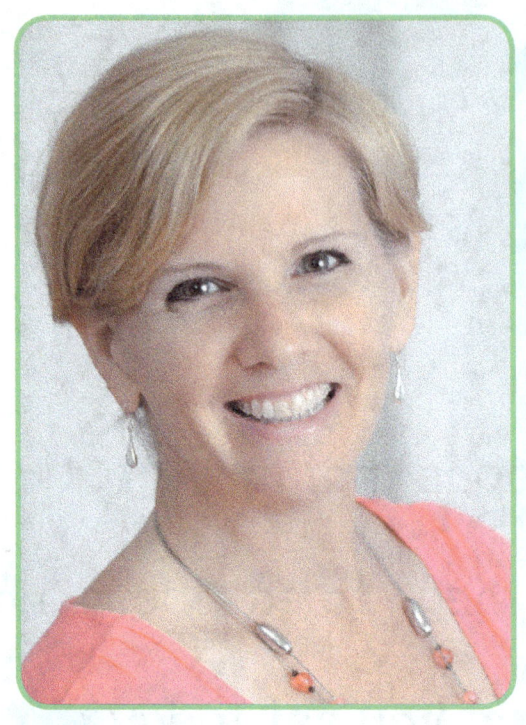

Tammy Letherer is a Chicago-based author and mother of three kids. She writes both fiction and non-fiction, and enjoys using her training as a Healing Touch Certified Practitioner to help children connect with their most authentic selves. Tammy could not live without peanut butter, and wonders when it will be classified a super food.

To learn about Tammy's other books, visit www.TammyLetherer.com.

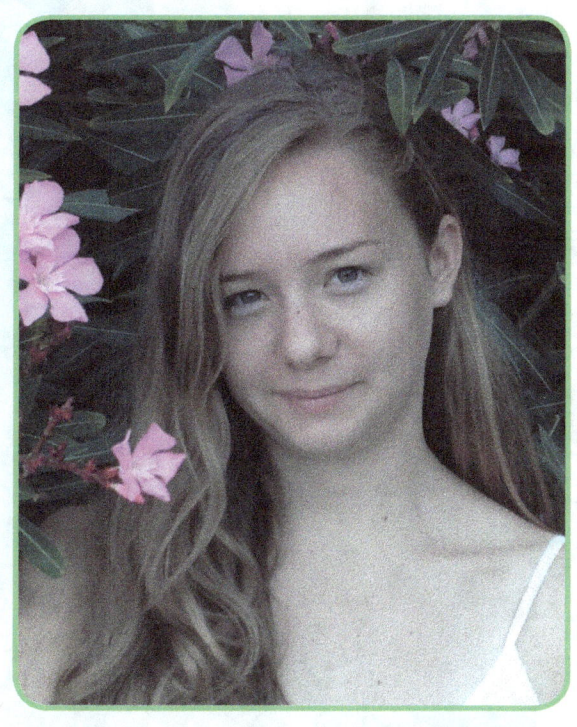

Catherine Hutchison grew up in Boulder, Colorado, where she learned to love nature, animals, and all things beautiful. She learned energy healing from her mother, Cynthia Hutchison, program director of the Healing Touch Program. She received a BA in Art from the University of Colorado, and loves to create energetic and spiritually-based artwork that inspires others to see the world in a different way. She enjoys circus arts and her favorite foods include blueberries and artichoke hearts (not together). This is her first illustrated book.